YOUR KNOWLEDGE HAS VALUE

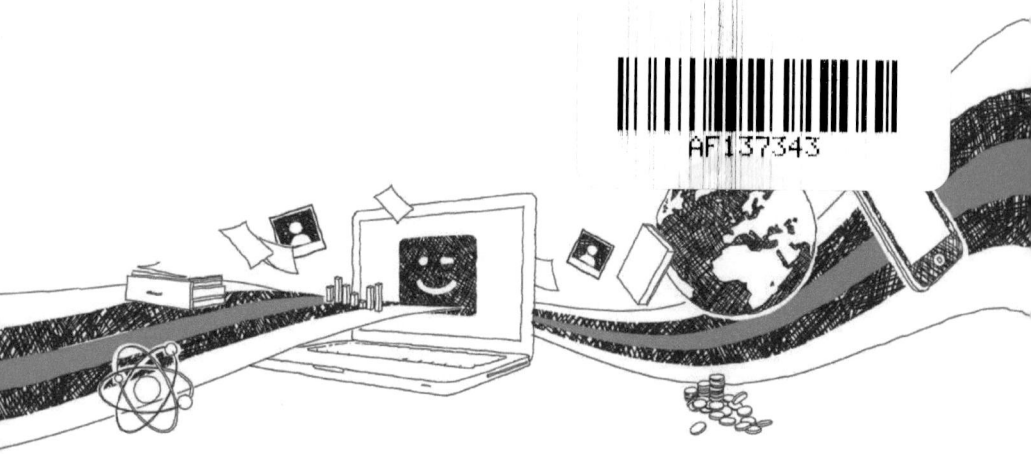

AF137343

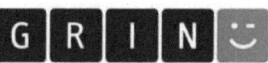

An Overview of the One Health Approach in Ethopia. Applications and Challenges

Isayas Asefa

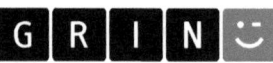

Bibliographic information published by the German National Library:

The German National Library lists this publication in the National Bibliography; detailed bibliographic data are available on the Internet at http://dnb.dnb.de.

ISBN: 9783346635945
This book is also available as an ebook.

© GRIN Publishing GmbH
Nymphenburger Straße 86
80636 München

Print and binding: Books on Demand GmbH, Norderstedt, Germany
Printed on acid-free paper from responsible sources.

The present work has been carefully prepared. Nevertheless, authors and publishers do not incur liability for the correctness of information, notes, links and advice as well as any printing errors.

GRIN web shop: https://www.grin.com/document/1192276

ONE HEALTH APPROACH IN ETHIOPIA: ITS APPLICATIONS AND CHALLENGES-OVERVIEW

SUMMARY

With the human population increment and inflate across the Planet, the interconnectedness of people, animals, and our surroundings becomes more significant and impactful. On the other hand, complications with worldwide environmental change, global health, antibiotics resistant pathogens, food safety, and emerging and re-emerging zoonotic diseases present variety of the foremost complex challenges to the health of the earth population. As separate disciplines cannot address these issues in isolation, and thus the potential economic, health, and environmental consequences of inaction are enormous. This review aimed toward sightseeing diversity of the applications and challenges of One health approach. One Health offers an inexpensive solution by recognizing the interconnected nature of human, animal, and ecosystem health in an attempt to reinforce health and environmental policy, expand knowledge base, improve health care training and delivery, identify and address upstream solutions to public health challenges. This idea is founded on an awareness of the most opportunities that exist to protect public health through policies aimed toward preventing and controlling pathogens at the interface between humans, animals, and thus the environment. One Health can also enhance strategies for sustainable development, especially in areas, where health issues are relevant to threatened wildlife populations, people, and animals. Despite its role in healthcare, operationalizing the concept of One Health requires overcoming many barriers including; difficulty in changing the mindset of health care providers from one among disease care to at least one of medicine, general lack of awareness, and wish for education of physicians about one health. In developing nations, the shortage of resources and informed personnel creates difficulty in establishing networks between animal, human and environmental health professionals. Even so, Challenges like monetary restrictions and lack of easy information exchange exist, it's critically important to develop this collaborative, cross-sectoral approach through that specialize in specific investment in governance, particularly with reference to the allocation of public and personal resources.

Keywords: *Applications; Challenges; Ethiopia: One health; Zoonotic diseases*

Inhalt

1. INTRODUCTION

One Health program is the concept that the health of the animal, human, and the viability of ecosystems are inseparably connected. The importance of the program is increasing as the enlargement of human and animal populations, ecological changes due to human impact and climate variations, and technological advancements facilitating global human, animal, and product movements have resulted in an increased risk of disease transmission between animals and people. It holds the idea that a disease problem impacting the health of humans, animals, and the environment can only be solved through improved communication, cooperation, and collaboration across disciplines and institutions (United States Department of Agriculture, 2015).

There are slightly varying definitions of One Health, most are similar to the European Union definition: One health is an integrated approach to health that focuses on the interactions between animals, humans, and their diverse environments. It encourages collaborations, synergies, and cross-fertilization of all professional sectors and actors in general whose activities may have an impact on health (European Union, 2015). One health recognizes that understanding these interactions and interdependencies necessitates an integrated perspective (Zinsstag, 2011). It represents an approach for developing and sustaining broad trans-disciplinary collaboration for the early identification, prevention, and mitigation of health risks in humans, animals, and the environment. This concept promotes a whole of society approach by incorporating human medicine, veterinary medicine, public health, and environmental information when developing policy and determining interventions to address current challenges threatening today's globalized world (HPED, 2011).

According to WHO, one or more new infectious diseases have emerged each year since the 1970s (WHO, 2007). The majority of these have been Zoonoses; diseases caused by pathogens that can be transmitted between animals and humans with more than three-quarters originating from wildlife (Jones *et al.*, 2008). Such diseases represent over 60% of all infectious organisms known to be pathogenic to humans (Food and Agriculture Organization, 2011). Global disease events have highlighted the increasing effects of zoonotic pathogens on human and animal health (Taylor *et al.*, 2001). It has also become evident that changes in the environment including; agricultural intensification, population growth, climate change, and human encroachment into wildlife habitats are drivers for such zoonotic disease emergence (Daszak *et al.*, 2013) and that environmental contamination with toxic chemicals and other hazards threaten human and animal populations (Rabinowitz *et al.*, 2009).

One Health aims to improve health and well-being through the prevention of risks and the mitigation of the effects of crises that originates at the interface between humans, animals, and their various environments (One Heath Global Network, 2015). The Cause of treatment failure in animals and humans attributable to antimicrobial resistance arising from the use of antimicrobial agents in food-producing animals or companion animals is a serious concern for public health (Australian Commission on Safety and Quality in Health Care, 2013).

The challenge to be better prepared for natural and man-made disasters is a huge concern for all, but veterinarians are in a unique position to appreciate the implication of disasters on both human and animal communities (Jones, 2009).

The commonalities of human and veterinary medicine and the financial constraints that many governments presently facing are arguments in favor of the One Health One Medicine approach, while the status of thinking, education system, administrative structures, and legislation hinder its application (Marsha and Tewodros, 2012). It was launched in Ethiopia in March, 2013 in collaboration with Jimma University with OHCEA Secretariat manager, and various delegates from local and international organizations (OHCEA, 2014). Its initiative draws national recognition and the team includes researchers, clinicians, and students from the Ohio State colleges of Nursing, Public Health, Medicine, and Veterinary Medicine. It focuses on health threats such as cervical cancer, rabies, neonatology, food, and environmental quality in East Africa (Gebreyes, 2015).

There is a lack of well-documented information regarding one health program in Ethiopia. Therefore; the objectives of this seminar paper are to review one health approach, its forthcoming applications, and challenges.

2. ONE HEALTH APPROACH

2.1. Origin and History of One Health Approach

Ever-growing human populations, striving 7 billion in 2011 (UNFPA, 2011), and the resulting environmental degradation from expanding land use, intensified agricultural and animal husbandry methods, and closer habitation between humans and both domesticated and wild animal species are recognized as key factors increasing shared risk across the animal-human-ecosystem interfaces (Sherman, 2010).

Generally, in the 20th century, three major movements were seen, all of which contributed largely to current thinking on one health approach. The first was the concept of 'One Medicine' which arose out of the work of Calvin Schwabe with Dinka in Sudan (Zinsstag *et al.*, 2011). Calvin Schwabe; the 'father of veterinary epidemiology' coined and reintroduced the concept of 'One Medicine' in his book Veterinary Medicine and Human Health in 1984, which argued that 'the critical needs of man include; the combating of diseases, ensuring enough food, adequate environmental quality and a society in which human values prevail' (Schwabe, 1984). His core idea echoed the 19[th]century physician Rudolf Virchow who believed that 'between animal and human medicine there are no dividing lines nor should there be' (Saunders, 2000). Schwabe renewed the basic principle that a more holistic approach to human, animal, and environmental health was needed to better protect the health of all (Schwabe, 1984).

The second movement was 'Ecosystem Health' or 'Eco-Health' which was adapted from ecology and environmental management to the improvement of human health and wellbeing. The third movement, which took the title of One Health, arose because of increasing concern of disease emergence at the interface between animals, humans, and ecosystems. Among a series of disease emergences of global importance in the 1990s triggering one health approach, Severe Acute Respiratory Syndrome (SARS), Avian influenza, and West Nile virus had strong participation from veterinary and, to a lesser extent, human public health (Nabarro, 2012).

In 1999, a series of themed conferences were organized by the Society for Tropical Veterinary Medicine and the Wildlife Diseases Association under the banner 'Working together to promote global health'. The second of these conferences held in 2001 in Pilanesberg, South Africa, addressed issues at the domestic animal and wildlife interface relating to disease control, conservation, sustainable food production, and emerging diseases (Gibbs and Bokma, 2002). This meeting is considered as key to the early development of One Health (Lee and Brumme, 2013).

In 2007, a vision supporting the concept of OH was adopted by The American Veterinary Medical Association and the American Medical Association that ended with the formation of the One Health Initiative task force. This brought together USA human and animal health agencies, medical doctors, and Veterinarians. Within the same year, the National Strategy for Pandemic Influenza and its Implementation Plan resulted in several International Ministerial Conferences that involved the United Nations' the FAO, the OIE, and the WHO. It has also gained ground throughout the USA government, led by the president's new initiatives for coordination and collaboration on national security and global development policy (United States Department of Agriculture, 2015).

1

2.2. History and establishment of One Health in Ethiopia

One Health was launched in Ethiopia on March 16, 2013, at Harmony Hotel in collaboration with Jimma University with the OHCEA Secretariat manager and various delegates from local and international organizations. Keynote address was delivered through delegates of the ministry of health and ministry of agriculture and both expressed the need for a One Health approach in the control and understanding of emerging diseases. The issue of collaboration was not new for the Ethiopian system since the two ministries in particular and other relevant disciplines were working together to address different health problems such as the case of unknown liver disease in the Western part of the Tigray region and avian influenza. They also said that the need for working together is a timely approach not only to solve communicable diseases but also the non-communicable diseases which affect both livestock and human beings (Gebreyes et al., 2014).

Furthermore, all representatives from governmental and private organizations appreciated OHCEA activities in Ethiopia so far and emphasized the need to consider the following points: focusing on advocacy of OH approach through creating more awareness forums to bring attitude change and get the buy-in of policymakers, working on a way of registering OHCEA in Ethiopia, and formulating short and long term goals at the national level, strengthening national committee and revising the existing membership to include all relevant OH stakeholders, soliciting funds or grants to make the present project sustainable after the current funding period expires, preparation of national strategic plan based on organized and well-designed assessment tool to know the gaps in various institutions/ organizations, documenting and sharing the lessons learned from previous ways of fighting pandemic threats in the form of success stories, working on gender issue to address zoonotic diseases (OHCEA, 2014).

2.2.1. One health initiation in Ethiopia

In Ethiopia, the One Health initiative draws national recognition. The team includes researchers, clinicians, and students from the Ohio State colleges of Nursing, Public Health, Medicine, and Veterinary Medicine, who focus on health threats such as cervical cancer, rabies, neonatology, and food and environmental quality in East Africa. The partnership has helped to install a capacity-building environment for faculty and students, created reciprocal adjunct faculty appointments, conducted workshops and field training through the One Health Summer Institute, and increased opportunities for students. The partnership integrates academics and practitioners from Ohio State, Ethiopia, and East African countries to leverage their knowledge, skills, and resources to contribute to improving biological and economic health in developed and underdeveloped countries (Gebreyes, 2015).

2.2.2. Objectives of one health program

Meeting new global challenges head-on through collaboration among multiple professions: Veterinary Medicine, human medicine, environmental, wildlife, and public health. Acting with professionalism in everything that they do, providing high-quality education and participating in life-long learning; providing outstanding veterinary medical care, building interdisciplinary teams both within and outside the college to address the needs of students, college community, patients, and society; seeking partnerships to bring together individual knowledge and talents from across the college, university, and profession; actively participating in activities and university initiatives that impact our college, maintaining respect and appreciation for areas outside of our individual

2

interests and expertise, creating a safe environment for engaging in candid and respectful discussion of differing opinions, recognizing that people matter, valuing the contributions that individuals, in different roles, bring to achieve the vision and missions (Second OHCEA International One Health Conference, 2015).

Removing artificial boundaries that divide us, understanding and utilizing all of our strengths so that each person has the opportunity and tools to achieve their full potential, working to provide and accept honest and constructive feedback, maintaining an attitude of flexibility and adaptability, avoiding the 'it's always been done that way' trap, being open to having our opinions challenged constructively; looking for new opportunities to lead the profession in education, discovery, patient care, and public service, proactively responding to and providing creative solutions to address the needs of our society (Gebreyes, 2015).

2.2.3. The scope of one health

The scope of One Health is impressive, broad, and growing. Some of the dimensions defining the scope of the concept are agro and bio-terrorism, antimicrobial resistance; basic, translational, and biomedical research, clinical, comparative, and conservative medicine, diagnosis; surveillance, control, and response to chemicals, toxicants, and radioactive substances. Further, it encompasses entomology, ethics (ensuring safe food and water supply, public policy regulatory enforcement); global trade and commerce, conservation of the natural resource and disaster preparedness; health communications and outreach, environmental health; infectious disease, ecology; integrated systems for detection of land use and production systems. Moreover, microbiology education, occupational health; public awareness and communications, scientific discovery and knowledge creation; support of biodiversity, training veterinarians, and environmental health professionals are to name a few (American Veterinary Medical Association, 2008).

2.3. Principles of One Health Approach

One Health recognizes the inseparable linkage of human, livestock, companion animal, wildlife, and environmental health implying an added value to the health and wellbeing of humans, animals, and the environment (Zinsstag *et al.*, 2011). This concept is more expanded compared to One Medicine that stated 'human and veterinary medicine share a common body of knowledge in anatomy, physiology, pathology and the origins of diseases in all species' (Schwabe, 1984), and thereby recognizing the mutual benefits available through the connection of veterinary medicine and human health. So, One Health is different from One Medicine in that ecosystem health is added into the animal-human interface to incorporate the environment, as well as wildlife populations, and recognize that sustainable development and continued human and animal health are dependent on healthy surrounding ecosystems (Zinsstag, 2011).

This new concept is the function of the collaborative efforts and communication of multiple disciplines working to attain optimal health of people, animals, and the environment. One Health is an integrated strategy that involves the cumulative works of veterinary medicine, human medicine, environmental science, and public health (Samuel *et al.*, 2013). More recently, it is defined as the collaborative effort of multiple health science professions together with their related disciplines and institutions working locally, nationally, and globally to attain optimal health for people, domestic animals, wildlife, plants, and our environments (One Health Commission, 2015).

Improving health and well-being through the prevention of risks and the mitigation of the effects of crises that originate at the interface of humans, animals, and their various environments is the aim of the One Health Approach. To promote this multi-sectoral and collaborative approach and a whole society approach to health hazards, a systemic change of perspective in the management of risks is crucial (One Health Global Network, 2015). Meeting new global challenges head-on through collaboration among multiple professions: Veterinary Medicine, human medicine, environmental health, wildlife, and public health (AVMA, 2008).

3. APPLICATIONS OF ONE HEALTH APPROACH

Weakening government public health services and stagnating public health and veterinary budgets in many countries have seriously limited disease surveillance and other preventive operations (World Bank, 2009). Global emerging livestock markets and rapidly changing socio-economic conditions, especially in parts of Asia and Africa (Herrero *et al.*, 2010), have led to the worrying development of 'flashpoints' of zoonotic disease emergence. These regions are increasingly compromised when it comes to public health. Their populations are already challenged by a host of endemic zoonosis that contributes to poverty both directly, through their impact on human and livestock health, and indirectly, through their cumulative effects on food and economic security (WHO, 2009).

Old-style farming practices continue alongside innovative methods to increase livestock productivity, but weak regional regulatory systems and national disease control responses often mean that rapidly changing systems have the potential to not only cause the emergence and re-emergence of zoonotic infections but also, more importantly, to further alienate already marginalized smallholder populations, as seen in the Avian influenza outbreaks in Asia (Scooness, 2010). Humans living close to and/or having frequent contact with wild animals and livestock, and sharing the same ecosystem with them, all contribute to the emergence of zoonotic disease. A lack of community awareness, the absence of effective surveillance in humans and animals, and limited access to human health care and veterinary services serve to aggravate the risk (Maudlin, 2009).

One Health approach that enables the management of both emerging and endemic zoonotic diseases may offer a practical and cost-effective route to poverty alleviation, by simultaneously addressing ecosystems management, animal and human health surveillance, and community participation in disease risk mitigation (Godfroid *et al.*, 2013).

A combined effort from the part of medical practitioners, veterinarians as well as ecologists, and environmentalists are requisite in implementing the concept which still remains as a theoretical idea (Conrad, 2013). The 5 C's (consensus, collaboration, cooperation, coordination, and commitment) for implementing the one health includes consensus among stakeholders, collaboration among professionals, cooperation among interdisciplinary groups, coordination among partner agencies, and commitment (political and financial) by donors, partners, organizations and governments. Financial assistance of US $1.3 billion allocated for one health per year till 2020 for low- and middle-income nations (World Bank, 2010).

3.1. One Health-From Veterinary Perspective

The three strongly interlinked pillars of veterinary medicine are Animal health, public health, and Animal welfare. The Core domains of Veterinary Public Health are diagnosis, monitoring, surveillance, and epidemiology; control and prevention of zoonosis; food safety; biomedical research; management of wildlife populations and management of public health emergencies (Federation of Veterinarians of Europeans, 2007). The following are veterinary perspectives in One Health Program:

3.1.1. The conservation of wildlife

Among existing and emerging pathogens affecting humans, over 60% originates from animals; of those, 75% comes from wildlife (FAO, 2011). Human intrusion into wildlife habitats invites these infectious agents to become pathogens for human populations. It is important to identify the routes by which these agents find their way to the human host and to understand their impact on the animals that serve as the primary and intermediate hosts. Veterinarians are in a unique position to organize their backgrounds and understanding of animal diseases to identify, manage and control these diseases (Jones, 2009). While human and domestic animal diseases do sometimes affect wildlife, pathogens that are transmitted from wildlife to humans, often through domestic animals, are considerably more numerous. These include HIV, Ebola, SARS, H5N1 Avian influenza, Nipah and Hantaviruses, Lyme disease, Crimean-Congo hemorrhagic fever, Tick encephalitis, and West Nile virus (Cleaveland *et al.*, 2001).

3.1.2. The safety of food

The meeting of people, animals, and our environment has created a new dynamic one in which the health of each group is inseparably interconnected. The challenges associated with this dynamic are demanding, profound, and unique. While the demand for animal-based protein is expected to increase by 50% by 2020, animal populations are under heightened pressure to survive, and further loss of biodiversity is highly probable (Delgado *et al.*, 1999). It's increasingly important to provide safe and adequate food and water for the world as the global population to the brink of seven billion consumers. Veterinarians have the expertise to address food production practices, ecosystem management, and microbial contamination problems associated with food safety (Scott, 2008).

3.1.3. Catastrophe alertness

The challenge to be better prepared for natural and man-made disasters is a huge concern for all, but veterinarians are in a unique position to appreciate the implication of disasters on both human and animal communities. Currently, the overwhelming majority of disaster relief efforts are targeted only, but veterinarians understand a complex link between humans and animals. Drawing on their knowledge of animal epidemiology, health husbandry, and behaviors, veterinarians can uniquely contribute to improving the quality of life for both animals and humans in the event of a disaster (Jones, 2009).

3.1.4. Control of zoonotic diseases

The concept of One Health mainly focuses on the control of various infectious diseases that can be transmitted among and between animals, humans, and the environment. Different indications show the occurrence of infectious diseases in different forms will continue to be significant global events (Graham *et al.*, 2008).

A large majority of these infectious diseases are caused by microbes that have zoonotic importance. Over 70% of human pathogens originate from animals for instance: Anthrax, Influenza, BSE, Brucellosis, Campylobacteriosis, Lyme Borreliosis, Rabies, Toxoplasmosis,

Tuberculosis, Salmonellosis, Leishmaniasis, Echinococcosis (Federation of Veterinarians of Europeans, 2007). About 75% of emerging infectious diseases over the past decade have been caused by pathogens originating from animals or their products. Veterinarians find themselves on the front lines in recognizing, diagnosing, and responding to these diseases (Clifford, 2009).

Most of these factors have contributed to establish a suitable condition and possibilities for the microbes to flare up every time and create new niches. These microbial, environmental, natural, and manmade changes are occurring very quickly worldwide and establish new beachheads in the populations of people, animals and are also invading our environment where they are inducing new pathogenic conditions (Coker *et al.*, 2011) as indicated in figure 1 below. The health of the animals, hygiene, and safety of food of animal origin represent growing and difficult challenges that clearly fall into a new global health agenda for animal production and food supply (Gebreyes *et al.*, 2014).

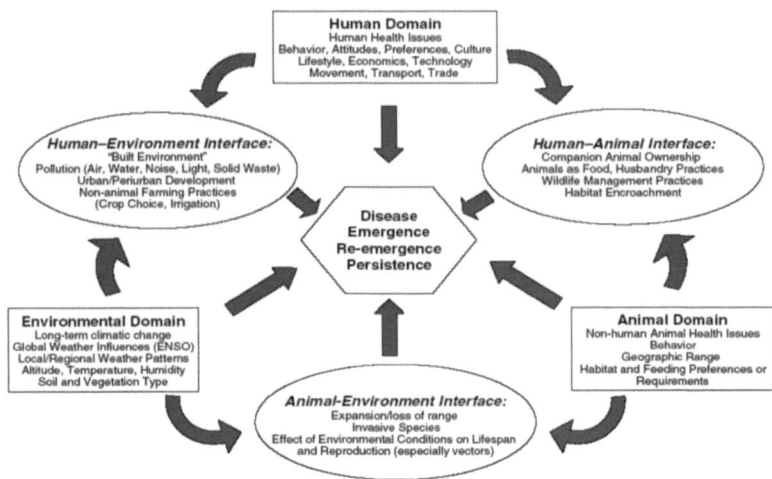

Figure 1. Major contributing factors for the emergence of emerging and re-emerging zoonotic diseases. Source: (Treadwell, 2008).

3.1.5. Environmental health

The environment includes "all of the physical, chemical and biological factors and processes that determine the growth and survival of an organism or a community of organisms". Another concept, the Ecosystem, is "comprised of all of the organisms and their physical and chemical environment within a specific area" (Christensen, 2012). Fundamentally, the environment affects how organisms live, thrive, and interact and must be considered to achieve optimal health for people and animals (Maller *et al.*, 2008). In general, human and animal well-being relies on the integrity of ecosystems. Ecosystems underpin processes essential to our survival, known as ecosystem services. These services include supporting services (nutrient cycling, soil formation, primary production); regulating services (climate and flood regulation, disease buffering, water purification); provisioning services (food, water, fuel); and cultural services (aesthetic, spiritual, mental health) that make the persistence of human and animal life possible (United Nations Millennium Ecosystem Assessment, 2005). Even though Ecosystems can maintain healthy populations, mismanagement or rapid alteration due to human pressure leads to increasing challenges to the maintenance of healthy ecosystems, including climate change, deforestation and intensification of agricultural systems, freshwater depletion, and resultant biodiversity loss which can also be associated with disease emergence (Myers and Patz, 2009).

3.1.6. Antibiotic resistance

Antibiotics are used widely to prevent or treat disease in food animals. The major part of the usage is for the prevention of disease, and their use has become an integral part of modern industrialized food animal production, to the extent where nearly all feed for growing animals is supplemented with antimicrobials in various doses, ranging from so-called "sub-therapeutic concentrations" to full therapeutic doses. It is estimated that the volumes of antimicrobials used in food animals exceed the use in humans worldwide, and nearly all the classes of antimicrobials that are used for humans are also being used in food animals, including the newest classes of drugs such as third- and fourth-generation cephalosporins, fluoroquinolones, glycopeptides, and streptogramins (Aarestrup *et al.*, 2008).

The public health consequences of zoonotic antibiotic-resistant pathogens are always difficult to assess for several reasons: the epidemiology is highly complex because it involves complex production and distribution systems of animals and food, it involves the spread of bacterial clones as well as resistant genes, and, finally, the impact on public health includes increased morbidity and mortality and higher costs of treatment of disease. Evidence shows that the amount and pattern of non-human usage of antimicrobials impacts the occurrence of resistant bacteria in animals and on food commodities and thereby human exposure to these resistant bacteria. The food-borne route is the major transmission pathway for resistant bacteria and resistant genes from food animals to humans, but other routes of transmission also exist (FAO *et al.*, 2003).

4. CHALLENGES OF ONE HEALTH APPROACHES

Effective long-term public-private partnership (PPP) is necessary for the success and sustainability of the program. Monitoring, evaluation, and implementation of this program will be a complex task, given the involvement of a large number of partners, wide geographical coverage, and multidisciplinary approach. Successful adoption of the program would have the advantage of Pooling and thus more efficient use of expertise and financial resources to address a common problem across the three health systems, the synergy of different institutional perspectives and experiences. Coordinated multi-sectorial action that brings together those working on human, animal, and ecosystems health is needed to address the impact of diseases occurring at the animal–human–ecosystems interface (FAO, 2008).

One health approach is getting worldwide acceptance as a strategic and all-inclusive approach in fighting global health problems which the connections between humans, animals, and the environment. In addition to these economic, cultural, and physical factors that influence health also recognized by the approach. The emerging and re-emerging diseases were driven by several factors. Thus, includes genetic and biological factors (microbial adaptation to macro-and microenvironmental changes, changes in host susceptibility to infection) environmental factors (climatic change, ecosystems change, and human and animal demography and densities changes), and socioeconomic and political factors (Increasing international travel and trade, social inequality, poverty, famine, changes in economic development and land use). According to the Institute of Medicine report, these factors were referred to as driving forces for the emergence of new zoonotic diseases and creates a favorable condition for the microbial population to appear (Smolinski et al, 2003).

4.1. Socio-Political Challenges

Application of one health concept will be challenged with socio-political issues because of people's belief and attachment with rights and freedoms even though they cannot pay sacrifice for the concern of others. For this reason, zoonotic disease control and prevention policy-making depend on individual behavior than factors that drive disease emergence/re-emergence (Rosella et al., 2013). Egoism, perceptions, short-term solutions, populism, and avoiding argument are characteristics of politics that result in challenges for emerging zoonotic disease prevention and control policymaking and affect the development of effective strategies for addressing EIDs (Degeling et al., 2015).

4.2. Budgetary Constraints

Sharing finances being constrained by low and unequal budget allocations. The human health sector generally has significantly more human and financial resources available for disease control activities than environmental or animal health agencies. Moreover, the relationship between staff salaries and recurrent costs to enable the services to operate has declined, leaving limited flexible spending for all services. This has been well documented for the veterinary services; in particular for sub-Saharan Africa (World Bank, 2009). The challenge of capacity can be an issue for government bodies as not all countries can support a One Health agenda. This lack of resources and informed personnel may prove difficult in establishing networks between animal, human, and environmental health professionals (FAO et al, 2008).

4.3. Unproductive Information Sharing

National public health authorities often use different disease reporting procedures and communication channels than the veterinary services. Despite the importance of understanding the life cycle of pathogens in humans, and in both domestic and wild animals, most national and international health organizations monitor, and can only generate information on, human or domestic animal disease but not both together (Kuehn, 2006). Professionals within the One Health field argue that there is a disconnection between professions working within the framework, specifically those from veterinary and medical communities. The inability to effectively coordinate professional services could jeopardize communication and surveillance regarding emerging zoonotic disease and curb the opportunity for collaboration in other interconnected matters of public health concern (Zinsstag et al, 2011).

4.4. Challenge of Managing Wildlife Ecosystem

The ecosystem changes due to driving forces that can alter the state of well-being and leads change to the interaction between human and animal populations (Smolinski, 2003). It is important to identify the routes by which the wild animal reservoirs agent found their way to the human host and their impact on the animals that serve as the primary and intermediate hosts (Jackson, 2015). It is more difficult to monitor diseases in wildlife due to afraid of aggressive wild animals, lack of knowledge and experience, inadequate financial recourse, and lack of road. Wild animals are not constrained by boundaries and can extend over large distances. This is particularly for migratory birds or mammals which seasonally move across continents or vast oceans which cause the spreading of disease (Singer et al., 2003). The declines and disappearances of different wildlife species are due to the disease of a certain pathogen. Practical difficulties can exist in determining the mortality rates because of dispersal after a disease outbreak. It can also be difficult for many different reasons to find and count both sick and dead wild animals (Jackson, 2015).

4.5. Problem of Working Together

Collaboration, involving different disciplines both within and beyond the health sciences to address transnational health issues and solutions. One Health approach offers an even broader multi-systems perspective on health means and the inclusion of a wider range of expertise to include areas of academic specialization (ICOPHAI, 2011). Conceptual and methodological differences between professionals of veterinary and human medicines are the most substantial challenges faced by collaborative working across the globe (Barlow et al., 2011).

Scientific knowledge and technical achievement are more important for the success of the One Health approach. To develop more holistic and diverse understandings of health across cultures, species, ecosystems, and local communities there are a lot of global challenges (Barlow et al., 2011). Clearly involving community members in health projects is essential for planning interventions that do not accidentally have negative health effects due to a failure to take into account the complexity and specificity of local conditions. Engaging communities inland-use decisions and approaches to disease control should be part of an integrated One Health approach (Anderson, 2004).

4.6. Ethical Concern

Active zoonotic disease combating policy relies on its implementation context and especially on its alignment with stakeholder and public principles (Mackenzie *et al.,* 2013). Like in modern liberalism there should be a few agreements over what is in the community interest and an understanding of the values which sustain it is required for the achievement of zoonotic disease prevention. However, this is in particular what has been missing in epidemics where fracture lines differences and value conflicts have become noticeable (Degeling *et al.*, 2015).

Other occurrence happens that stakes are high, evidence and the implication of actions are uncertain, the situation is complex and resources are limited but where decisions need to be made its ethical differences are exposed to challenge (Singer *et al.,* 2003.) This difference could be due to beliefs that deal with ecological and environmental issues that can be mismatched with the significance of people's connection to public goods, protection of individual and animal welfare (Degeling *et al.,* 2015). This condition results in adverse costs of public fear, doubt, misinformation, and disobedience to public health directives (Davies, 2010). Successful response of outbreaks in a One Health approach wants to address the above stated ethical concerns. To do this successfully diverging values and logic must be negotiated to realize effective, sustainable, and just solutions by considering the public interest as an apriority task (Rosella *et al.,* 2013).

5. CONCLUSION AND RECOMMENDATIONS

Generally speaking, the One Health approach urges synergistic ways to deal with the assortment, investigation, and understanding of a wide scope of knowledge to thwart and react to the quickly changing environment and its effects on the health of humans and animals' networks. This methodology must be effective if it jams organizations across different expert areas and partakes investors inside the humans, animals, and environment classes. It motivates further developed community-oriented contribution opportunities for counteraction and reaction to diseases. Regardless of the huge and developing assemblage of identification supporting its helpfulness, the extraordinary greater part of clinical instruction, clinical practice, improvement projects, and examination keep on working inside disciplinary limits. This absence of take up of the OH approach ascribes to lacking identification to convince professionals and leaders.

Besides, perplexing public health difficulties will keep on arising which must be endeavored through the utilization of One Health.

Given the above deduction the ensuing suggestions are frequently sent:

i. Spilling over doubt inside the overall humans and animal health setup reasonable with the staggering thought of emerging and resurging affliction threats to humans, animal, and untamed life.

ii. Giving off a consolation agenda, through the foundation of joint financial agendas of the administrations, and therefore the arrangement of extraordinary subsidizing instruments for One Health exercises.

iii. Enactment ought to be ready and executed to advance the One Health approach through disease announcing and dynamic cycles.

iv. The instructive program must be created, specifically at the college level that incorporates humans, animals, and environmental health and acquaints the standards of One Health.

v. Accordingly, capacity building via preparing health experts, awareness creation to the community through health extension workers, and advancing community health programs in the One Health approach required.

6. REFERENCES

Aarestrup, F., Wegener, H., Collignon, P., 2008. Resistance in bacteria of the food chain; Epidemiology and control strategies. Expert Review of Anti-Infective Therapy, **6:** 733–750.

American Veterinary Medical Association (AVMA), 2008. One Health: a new professional imperative; One Health Initiative Task Force: Final Report Pp 3.

American Veterinary Medical Association and Western Veterinary Congress, 2008. One World One Health, One Medicine. President's Messages, 49:1063.

Anderson, 2004. Natural histories of infectious disease: ecological vision in 20th century Biomedical Science. Osiris, **19:** 39-61.

Australian Commission on Safety and Quality in Health Care, 2013. Antimicrobial Resistance: A Report of the Australian One Health Antimicrobial Resistance Colloquium, Australian Government.

Barlow, J, Ewers, R, Anderson, L, Aragao, L, Baker, T.,2011. Using learning networks to understand complex systems, a case study of biological, geophysical, and social research in the Amazon. Biological Reviews of the Cambridge Philosophical Society: 86(**2**): 457-474.

Christensen, N., 2012. The environment and you, Boston, Addison Wesley.

Clifford, D and Coppolillo, P, 2009. One Health Approach to Address Emerging Zoonoses: Health in action, 6:1-5. Website: www.plolsmedicine.org. Accessed on April 11, 2019.

Coker, R., Rushton, J., Mounier-Jack, S., Karimuribo, E. and Lutumba, P., 2011. Towards a conceptual framework to support One Health research for policy on emerging zoonosis. Lancet Infectious Diseases, **11:** 326–331.

Conrad P, Meek L, Dumit J.,2013. Operationalizing a One Health approach to global health challenges. Comparative Immunology: Microbial Infection Disease **36:** 211-216.

Daszak, P., Zambrana-Torrelio, C., Bogich, T., Fernandez, M., Epstein, J., Murray, K, 2013. Interdisciplinary approaches to understanding disease emergence: the past, present, and future drivers of Nipah virus emergence: Proceedings of the National Academy of Sciences USA; **110** (Supplement1): 3681–8.

Davies, S, 2010. What contribution can international relations make to the evolving global health agenda: International Affairs **86:** 43-65.

United Nations Millennium Ecosystem Assessment, 2005.

Myers, S, and Patz, J., 2009. Emerging threats to human health from global environmental change: Annual Review of Environment and Resources **34:** 223- 252.

Degeling, C, Johnson, J, Kerridge, I, Wilson, A, Ward, M., 2015. Implementing One Health Approach to Emerging Infectious Disease, Reflections on the socio-political, ethical, and legal dimensions. BMC Public Health 15: 1307.

Delgado, C, Rosegrant, M, Steinfeld, H, 1999. Livestock to 2020: The next food revolution. Food, Agriculture, and the Environment discussion paper 28. Washington DC, International Food Policy Research Institute.

European Union, 2015. One Health: addressing health risks at the interface between animals, humans, and their environments: International Journal of Circumpolar Health, **74.**

FAO, OIE, WHO., 2003: Joint FAO/OIE/WHO Expert Workshop on Non-Human Antimicrobial Usage and Antimicrobial Resistance: Scientific assessment; Geneva, Pp 1-20.

FAO, WHO, OEI, UNICEF., 2008. The World Bank, Contributing to One World-One Health. A strategic framework for reducing risks of infectious diseases at the animal-human–ecosystems interface. New York, NY: United Nations.

Federation of Veterinarians of Europeans, 2007. One Health: Pulling Animal Health and Public Health Together. Brussels.

Food and Agriculture Organization, 2008. Contributing to One World, One Health. A Strategic Framework for Reducing Risks of Infectious Diseases at the Animal-Human Ecosystems Interface.

Food and Agriculture Organization, 2011. One Health, Food, and Agriculture Organization of the United Nation Strategic Action Plan, Pp 3.

Gebreyes, W., 2015. Ethiopia One Health initiative draws national recognition. The Ohio State University College of Veterinary Medicine CVM Webmasterry Medical Center. 601 Vernon L. Tharp Street. Columbus, OH 43210.

Gebreyes, W., Dupouy, C., Newport, M., Oliveira, C., and Schlesinger, L., 2014. The Global One Health Paradigm: Challenges and Opportunities for Tackling Infectious Diseases at the Human, Animal, and Environment Interface in Low- Resource Settings. PLOS Neglected Tropical Diseases, **8**: e3257.

Gebreyes, W., Jean, D., Melanie, J., Celso, J., Larry, S., Yehia, M., Samuel, K., Linda, J., William, S., Thomas, W., Armando, H., Sylvain, Q., Rudovick, K., Berhe, T., Thomas, S., Michael, B., Prapas, P., Sumalee, B. and Lonnie, J., 2014. The Global One Health Paradigm: Challenges and Opportunities for Tackling Infectious Diseases at the Human, Animal, and Environment Interface in Low-Resource Settings. PLOS Neglected Tropical Diseases, **8**:1-6.

Gibbs, E., and Bokma, B., 2002. The domestic animal/wildlife interface: issues for disease control, conservation, sustainable food production, and emerging diseases, Annals of the New York Academy of Sciences, 969.

Godfroid, J., Al Dahouk, S., Pappas, G., Roth, F., Matope, G., Muma, J., Marcotty, T., Pfeiffer, D., and Skjerve, E., 2013. A 'One Health' surveillance and control of brucellosis in developing countries: Moving away from improvisation. Comparative Immunology, Microbial Infectious Disease, **36**: 241–248.

Graham, J, Leibler, J, Price, L, Otte ,J, Pfeiffer, D., 2008. The animal-human interface and infectious disease in industrial food animal production: rethinking biosecurity and biocontainment. Public Health Reports **123**: 282-299.

Herrero, M., Thornton, P., Notenbaert, A., Wood, S., Msangi, S., Freeman, H., Bossio, D., Dixon, J., Peters, M., van de Steeg, J., Lynam, J., Parthasarathy Rao, P., Macmillan, S., Gerard B., McDermott, J., Seré, C. and Rosegrant, M. (2010): Smart investments in sustainable food production: Revisiting mixed crop-livestock systems Science **327**: 822–825.

HPED networking event (Highly Pathogenic and Emerging and re-emerging Diseases), 2011. Workshop report. Linking the actors of the EU-Asia Regional One Health Programme; 18-19 January; Bangkok, Thailand: European Commission, European Union.

ICOPHAI, 2011. First International Congress on Pathogens at the Human-Animal Interface (ICOPHAI). Addis Ababa, Ethiopia. Accessed on 6 April 2019.

Jackson, S, 2015. Economic Benefits of a One Health approach. The World Bank, Report No: ICR00003260, Implementation Completion and Results Report on the European Commission Avian and Human, Influenza Trust Fund (EC-AHI) Pp. 2.

Jones, E., 2009. One Health Commission Formed to Promote Collaboration Across Human, Animal, and Environmental Health Sciences: One Health Commission..

Jones, K., Patel, N., Levy, M., Storeygard, A., Balk, D., Gittleman, J., and Daszak, P. 2008. Global trends in human emerging infectious diseases. Nature, **451**: 990-993.

Kuehn, B., 2006. "Animal-Human Diseases Targeted to Stop Pandemics Before They Start." JAMA, **295:** 1987–1989.

Lee, K. and Brumme, Z., 2013. Operationalizing the One Health approach: the global governance challenges. Health Policy and Planning, **28**: 778–785.

Mackenzie, S, Jeggo, M, Daszak, P, Juergen A., 2013. One Health, The Human- Animal-Environment Interfaces in Emerging Infectious Diseases. Current Topics in Microbiology and Immunology **365**: 1-340.

Maller, C., Townsend, M., St Leger, L., 2008. Healthy parks, healthy people: the health benefits of contact with nature in a park context, second edition, Melbourne, Deakin University and Parks Victoria.

Marsha, C. and Tewodros, F., 2012. One Health One Medicine One World: Co-joint of Animal and Human Medicine with Perspectives. *Review on Veterinary World*, **5**: 238-243.

Maudlin, I., Eisler, M. and Welburn, S., 2009. Neglected and endemic zoonoses. Philosophical Transactions of

Nabarro, D., 2012. 'One Health: Towards safeguarding the health, food security and economic welfare of communities: Onderstepoort Journal of Veterinary Research, Article #450, **79:** 1-3.

Okello A, Gibbs E V, Ersmissen A, Welburn, S, 2011. One health and the neglected zoonoses: turning rhetoric into reality. Vet. Record **169**: 281-285.

One Health Centre of East Africa, 2014. One Health Launch Ethiopia. Jimma University.

One Heath Global Network, 2015. One Heath Program: World Health through Collaboration.

One Heath Global Network, 2015. One Heath Program: World Health through Collaboration; http/www.eeas.europa.eu/health/ and http/www.cdc.gov/one health.

Rabinowitz, P., Scotch, M., Conti, L., 2009. Human and animal sentinels for shared health risks. Veterinaria Italian, **45**: 23–24.

Rosella, L, Wilson, K, Crowcroi, N, Chu, A, Upshur, R., 2013. PandemicH1N1 in Canada and the use of evidence in developing public health policy analysis. Social Science Medicine **83**: 1-9.

Samuel, T., Shomaker, S., Shomaker, J., Eleanor, M., Green and Suzanne, M., 2013. One Health, A compelling convergence. *Academic Medicine*, **88**: 49-55.

Saunders, L., 2000. Commentary: Virchow's contribution to veterinary medicine: celebrated then, forgotten now. Veterinary Pathology, **37**: 199-207.

Schwabe, C., 1984. Veterinary Medicine and Human Health, Williams & Wilkins: Baltimore Third edition., Pp 1–680.

Scoones, I., 2010. Avian influenza: science, policy and politics. Routledge Earthscan, London.

Scott. C., 2008. The Intersection of Human, Animal and Environmental Health. Calvin Schwab One Health Project.

Second OHCEA International One Health Conference, 2015. Report of highlights, 7 December.

Sherman, D., 2010. A global veterinary medical perspective on the concept of One Health: focus on livestock. ILAR Journal; **51**: 281-7.

Singer, P, Benatar, S, Bernstein, M, Daar, A, Dickens, B., 2003. Ethics and SARS: lessons from Toronto. British Medical Journal **327**: 1342-1344.

Smolinski, M, Hamburg, M, Lederberg, J., 2003. Microbial Threats to Health: Emergence, Detection, and Response. National Academy Press, Washington, DC, USA.

Taylor, L., Latham, S., Woolhouse, M. 2001. Risk factors for human disease emergence. Philosophical Transactions of the Royal Society B: Biological Sciences, **356**: 983-9; the Royal Society B: Biological Sciences, **364**: 2777–2787.

United Nations Population Fund, UNFPA State of World Population, 2011. People and possibilities in a world of 7 billion. New York: UNFPA.

United States Department of Agriculture, 2015. One Health Program: Animal and Plant Health Inspection Service. Veterinary Service One Health

WHO, World Health Report, 2007. A Safer Future, Global Public Health Security in the 21st Century. Geneva, Switzerland: World Health Organization, Pp 2.

World Bank, 2009. Minding the Stock: Bringing Public Policy to Bear on Livestock Sector Development. Washington DC: Report No. 44010-Gramm Leach Bliley.

World Bank, 2010. Towards a One Health Approach for Controlling Zoonotic Diseases. In: People, Pathogens and Our Planet Report.50833-GLB.

Zinsstag, J., Schelling, E., Waltner-Toews, D. and Tanner, M., 2011. 'From one medicine" to "one health" and systemic approaches to health and well-being', Preventive Veterinary Medicine, **101**: 148–156.

YOUR KNOWLEDGE HAS VALUE

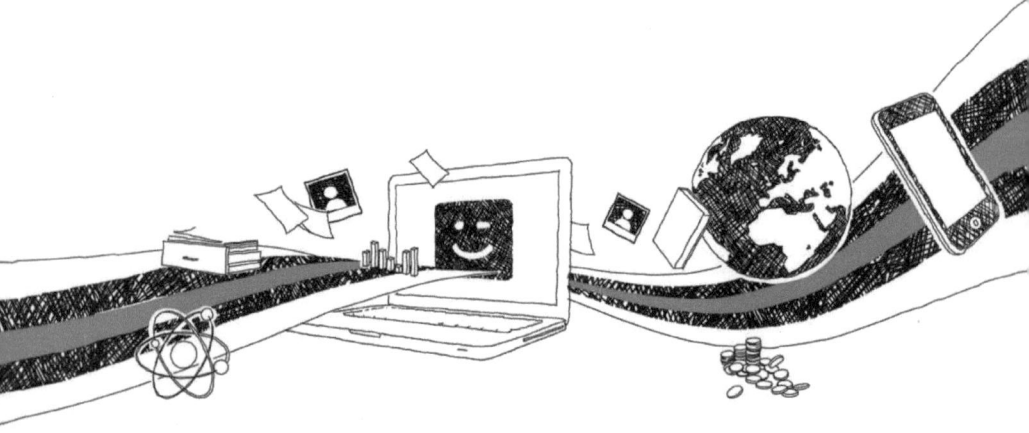

- We will publish your bachelor's and master's thesis, essays and papers

- Your own eBook and book - sold worldwide in all relevant shops

- Earn money with each sale

Upload your text at www.GRIN.com and publish for free

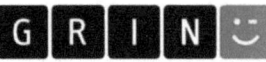